Unhealthy Politics

How professional, political, business and other self-interested lobbies have fought and are fighting attempts to enact a national health care program for all Americans.

By
Jerome F. Brazda

Airleaf Publishing

airleaf.com

ISBN: 1-60002-024-0

Contents

The Beginning

There are millions of non-elderly persons in the United States who have no health insurance; there is no legal guarantee that they will get whatever health care they may need. This is no accident. Progressive politicians since Teddy Roosevelt have attempted to make health care more widely available. But obstructive negative efforts by selfish interests have prevented substantial numbers of the nation's sick from getting the health care this great nation is capable of giving.

Harry and Louise are a fictional couple who appeared on television and radio, in 1993 and 1994, in a blatantly irresponsible advertising campaign by commercial health insurance companies opposed to any national health plan that might erode the billions of dollars they make off the nation's need for health care insurance for all. The Health Insurance Association of America, representing for-profit health insurers, invented the campaign to beat back President Bill Clinton's attempt to insure the uninsured. Having helped to accomplish that mission, they resurfaced when presidential candidates in the 2000 election campaign talked about bringing to the nation the universal guarantee of health care that Clinton, his wife, Hillary Rodham Clinton, and Vice President Al Gore were unable to do.

Harry and Louise are the tool of a well-heeled army of lobbyists who swarm Washington in a continuing campaign to, in effect, keep the uninsured uninsured—by the government, that is. It has been like that since President Franklin D. Roosevelt talked about including health security with Social Security, touching off the immediate opposition of organized medicine. President Lyndon B. Johnson battled the same entrenched interests to bring Medicare and Medicaid into existence in a classic political accomplishment over great odds.

The United States is the richest nation of earth, but one of the few without a national health plan. In an ironic twist, Dr. James Mongan, former Senate and White House aide now a health care executive, tells of the time that conservative icon Martin Feldstein, one of President Reagan's financial advisers, boasted in a conversation, "Maybe that's why" (we are the richest).

The lack of total coverage in this wealthy nation is a regrettable fact. Overcrowded hospital emergency rooms often are pressed to deliver care for the uninsured who have nowhere to go to be treated. Although this reality is being addressed by bits and pieces—such as changes in the historic Medicare law and fragmented attempts by the federal government to expand child health programs—health care in the United States is anything but a right such as free speech and protection from foreign invasion. To be assured of effective medical care Americans must be able to show they have some sort of insurance coverage. Otherwise they risk being broken financially or, in a sense, being left to die.

Opposition to any sort of federally backed universal health insurance program, in effect making health care a citizen's right, has been overwhelming. Any time a new program is suggested Washington veterans say, "Never mind who's for it; who's agin' it?" The negatives must be recognized before anyone can talk positively. This book is a long-time reporter's story of what has happened and how history is being repeated as political candidates try again and the negatives rise again. President Clinton saw the need and was elected in what was considered a mandate. But he failed in an inept effort in which the lessons of experience were not used.

If health care is to be a citizen's constitutional right, as it is in most other advanced societies, the federal government must guarantee its citizens health insurance coverage. Only a federal guarantee, not necessarily federal health insurance itself, as is so successfully used in Canada, can make coverage truly universal. Failure to learn from the past could result in another long wait while the ranks of the uninsured—and the sick—grow.

The Past as Prologue

Political interest in a government-driven compulsory health insurance plan for the United States has been fruitless for most of the 20th century. Initially more populous states began to look within their own borders to assure medical care for the sick and there was talk about health plans in legislatures. But no bills were enacted after opposition from conservative and medical sources began to appear.

The notion of universal medical care insurance began to assume national proportions in the United States after World War I. President Theodore Roosevelt had called for national health insurance and his Progressive Party adopted the idea as part of its platform in 1912. The American Association for Labor Legislation (AALL) was organized in 1906 and expanded for the next several years into a group of economists, attorneys, political scientists and others interested in social problems. Workmen's compensation laws resulted in many states as AALL began to look beyond the nation's healthcare needs.

In 1912, AALL established a Social Insurance Committee to look into the advisability of a standard health insurance bill. The bill would call for health care protection of all low income workers plus cash compensation and broad hospital and medical benefits to workers and their dependents. Several committee members were also members of the American Medical Association which, seeing that things were happening, named its own committee on Social Insurance. AMA, the American Hospital Association and the National Association of Manufacturers all viewed the proceedings with interest if not support and agreed to study the matter.

AALL initially concentrated on the principle of state action but, as its proposals expanded, the states mostly skirted the issue out of fear of the cost, deferring to a federal plan.

President Woodrow Wilson's developing liberalism had initially encouraged AALL to expand nationally, but Wilson, who had opposed social insurance earlier, eventually turned on Roosevelt's national health insurance plan.

In 1916, the secretary of AALL still reported opportunities for "compulsory health insurance legislation in this country in 1917." But negative, defensive lobbying developed as interested organizations realized what was being discussed.

A representative of Prudential Insurance Company of America resigned from the Committee on Social Insurance in 1916 when it endorsed compulsory medical insurance. Pharmaceutical companies, health and accident insurance companies and other professional and commercial interests expressed disfavor. Even great American labor leader Samuel Gompers of the AFL, apparently seeing a threat to his power as a benefits negotiator, attacked the idea of government health insurance.

AMA fluctuated in its support as AALL developed model bills for state or national plans. Various factions within the association began to direct their ire at Dr. Alexander Lambert, who served on the committee and appeared to favor compulsory health insurance. At its 1920 session in New Orleans, the AMA House of Delegates resolved that AMA "declares its opposition to the institution of any plan embodying the system of compulsory contributory insurance against illness or any other plan of compulsory insurance which provides for medical service to be rendered contributors or their dependants provided, controlled or regulated by any state or Federal government."

Two years later the House of Delegates voted opposition to the Sheppard-Towner bill, which provided federal subsidies for state-run child and maternal health programs, but the legislation passed nonetheless. The physicians testified against it as a threat of government interference in the private practice of medicine.

Several philanthropic foundations, such as Carnegie and Millbank, financed establishment of a Committee on the Costs of Medical Care, comprised of representatives of medical practice, public health interests and public representatives. The committee called for medical care through group practice to be paid for by insurance or taxation. The AMA'S response in the AMA Journal echoes through the ages:

"The alinement (sic) is clear—on the one side the forces representing the great foundations, public health officialdom, social theory—even socialism and communism—inciting to revolution; on the other side, the organized medical profession of this country urging an orderly evolution guided by controlled experimentation which will observe the principles that have been found through the centuries to be necessary to the sound practice of medicine."

In 1934, President Franklin D. Roosevelt acted on campaign promises to use government to erase the scourge of the Great Depression by naming a cabinet-level Committee on Economic Security to look into "all forms of social insurance." The list compiled by committee director Edwin E. Witte included health insurance in a laundry list of problems facing the nation.

To explore the idea of government health insurance Witte appointed Edgar Sydenstricker and I.S. Falk who had been members of the AALL Council on the Cost of Medical Care. The council recommended private health insurance as an answer but this still brought opposition from AMA members fearful of anything getting between the physician and patient, even third-party payers. Word that government health insurance was under discussion by the Roosevelt Administration drew strong protests from physicians. In fact, the President's own advisers were concerned that opposition from a group as strong as the medical profession might endanger Social Security.

Because the President had so much to lose, notes historian Peter A. Corning, the AMA's leverage was therefore increased; in effect the doctors could hold the whole Social Security bill hostage. Ironically, one private physician opposing the idea was the father-in-law of Roosevelt's son James.

After an intense battle among his advisers, heightened by a barrage of objections from physicians or their self-appointed representatives, the committee agreed with the President to recommend further study of the issue of national health insurance, implying the President favored the idea. Witte later wrote that the idea of more federal money for public health work was endorsed by the AMA. But the implications of the President favoring study of the feasibility of national health insurance so alarmed AMA it called the first emergency meeting of its House of Delegates since World War I. At the meeting delegates reversed their stand against all forms of health insurance and endorsed experimentation with voluntary plans under the control of county and state medical societies. It strongly condemned compulsory health insurance.

Nontheless the committee staff, completing the third leg of the stool, drafted a legislative proposal to be included in the Social Security bill as an amendment. The committee's report recommended: (1) federal financial aid for local public medical facilities and services, (2) cash benefits for temporary disability due to illness, (3) further study of the need for permanent disability benefits, and (4) federal subsidies for state-run health insurance programs that met "basic federal safeguards."

President Roosevelt decided, however, to hold off any inclusion of health in the Social Security bill. Witte wrote that "it was my original belief that it would probably be impossible to do anything about health insurance in a legislative way, due to the expected strong opposition of the medical profession." Presidential adviser Harry Hopkins was more interested in health insurance than any other social insurance, Witte said, "but also realized that this subject would have to be handled very gingerly."

Marathon discussions continued within the Roosevelt White House on the subject of national health insurance and the vitriolic and potentially damaging opposition of organized medicine. Witte wrote: "In the original Social Security bill there was one line to the effect that the Social Security Board should study the problem (regarding health insurance) and make a report thereon to Congress. That little line was responsible for so many telegrams to members of Congress that the entire Social Security program seemed endangered until the Ways and Means Committee unanimously struck (the line) out of the bill." Roosevelt, seeing no practical possibilities, chose to lay aside the committee report on health insurance.

AMA, through an editorial in the Nov. 24, 1934, Journal of the AMA, reported on the pressure behind its vehement opposition:

"The headquarters office of the American Medical Association has been besieged with telephone calls, telegrams and letters…some physicians are apparently opposed to all change and feel that the (AMA) should officially make itself felt in opposition to the entire program of the government." The editorial noted that while the House of Delegates "has repeatedly voiced its opposition to the socialization of medical practice, it indicated…its belief in properly controlled experimentation with new forms of medical practice." Still, any time action appeared possible on any proposal for a national medical care AMA was in opposition.

The Social Security Act finally was passed in 1935. There was no mention of healthcare in the new law, but several of its creators, notably Wilbur Cohen, remained in the government in various positions and eventually used the Social Security law as a vehicle for enactment of Medicare and Medicaid as Titles 18 and 19 in 1965.

As part of the Social Security Act, Congress authorized the Social Security Board to study further activities the government might undertake to assure the economic security of older citizens. As the board began to consider various needs for social legislation it did not consider health care. In the words of its chairman, Arthur Altmeyer: "Because of the strong opposition of the American Medical Association to health insurance the Social Security Board...did not give much attention to this subject during the first few months."

Roosevelt later decided he wanted no action on national health insurance in 1936, an election year. However, in 1935 he appointed an Interdepartmental Committee to Coordinate Health and Welfare Activities to oversee implementation of the Social Security Act and look for possible improvements. The committee took an interest in medical care. In 1937, a Technical Committee on Medical Care was named. The committee found a need for a medical care program and insurance against loss of wages because of illness.

A national health survey, conducted by the federal government in 1935-36, found the poor, especially people on relief, get sick more than the rich and stay ill longer. It also reported that much of the population had no way to pay for medical care. An American Association for Social Security was formed by Abraham Epstein to support the idea of government health insurance. Subsequently, Public Health Surgeon General Thomas Parran, Altmeyer and Hopkins held a private conference at the Brookings Institution to talk about a national health program. The group also included Josephine Roche of the Treasury Department which then included the Public Health Service, initially organized for health care needs of Coast Guardsmen.

The Technical Committee was expanded and assigned to work out a proposed national health program. It did so, then called a three-day conference at Washington's Mayflower Hotel to discuss the details. The program's five legislative proposals included: expansion of the maternal and child health and public health programs included in the original Social Security Act, federal grants-in-aid for hospital construction, grants to the states for direct medical programs for those on public assistance and the "medically indigent," grants to the states to encourage establishment of state-run health insurance programs, and establishment of a federal disability plan.

The conference, as much as anything, stimulated more controversy between the AMA and the Administration. Little else resulted.

The program was sent to Congress early in 1939 for study. Later that year, Democratic Senator Robert F. Wagner of New York introduced a bill of his own incorporating the national health program. Eleven days of hearings were held by the Committee on Education and Labor but no vote was taken. AMA, the American Hospital Association and the American Dental Association testified against it. Testifying for it were organized labor and several civic, welfare and agricultural groups.

By 1940 Roosevelt, faced with a growing international crisis and opposition to an unprecedented third term, saw Congressional Democrats, led by Southerners, line up with Republicans in a conservative coalition. He did not make national health care an issue in the campaign. The Wagner bill died in committee, but in 1943 as news from the war front became more favorable, allowing consideration of domestic issues, Wagner was joined by Sen. John Murray (D-Mont.) And Rep. John Dingell (D-Wis.). The triumvirate sponsored what became known as the Wagner-Murray-Dingell bill, a comprehensive social measure that included a national health program along with other benefits.

Roosevelt died before he could resume advocacy of a national health plan as he had been expected to do. But in November of 1945 new President Harry Truman sent a message to Congress endorsing Wagner-Murray-Dingell.

Truman asked for compulsory health insurance funded by payroll deductions. All Americans would be eligible for medical and hospital service. Truman pursued the idea with enthusiasm. His State of the Union message in 1947 called for national health insurance including support for mental health and hospital construction. But conservative opposition, particularly, from the AMA which was horrified by Truman's surprise election, was so strong that Truman was never able to further his ideas. After Truman's upset 1948 victory the AMA House of Delegates voted a special assessment of members "to resist the enslavement of the medical profession."

AMA was particularly startled by Truman's appointment of Oscar Ewing, a staunch supporter of national health insurance, to head the Federal Security Agency, the forerunner to the Social Security Administration. Ewing issued a report called "The Nation's Health, a Ten-Year Program: A Report to the President" that called for compulsory health insurance. The AMA responded by hiring for $1million (a lot of money then) a California political public relations firm, Whitaker and Baxter. The firm had helped the California Medical Association defeat Republican Gov. Earl Warren's proposal for a state compulsory health insurance program.

Truman had called for a national health plan financed by Social Security taxes. Clem Whitaker told a meeting of AMA leaders in Chicago early in 1949 that "Oscar Ewing, the great patent medicine man…apparently is grimly determined to bring socialized medicine from sick England to healthy America." The public campaign by Whitaker and Baxter was harsh worded and unrelenting. The firm resurfaced during AMA's battle against Medicare 15 years later.

Truman sought to appoint Ewing head of a cabinet-level Federal Security Agency but the proposal was defeated twice, first by the Senate, then by the House by an overwhelming margin, thanks largely to the typically intensive and negative lobbying by AMA. Truman finally gave up, writing years later it was one of his most bitter disappointments.

Although President Dwight D. Eisenhower did establish the Department of Health, Education and Welfare there was very limited interest in his administration in a national health plan. HEW Undersecretary Nelson Rockefeller, a more moderate Republican, was said to favor some form of national health care, but nothing surfaced from his office. Arthur Fleming, later Undersecretary, then Secretary of HEW, was interested in the public health but also was unable to find sympathy among administration officials.

During the Eisenhower years, however, Social Security advocate Wilbur Cohen joined with several Democratic senators, including John F. Kennedy, in support of a disability insurance program within Social Security. The AMA stoutly opposed the movement, warning members that disability insurance was the foot in the door for socialized medicine.

About that time Cohen and Kennedy aide Ted Sorenson proposed to Senator Kennedy a program of hospital insurance for the elderly under Social Security. It would take several years and unimaginable tragedy before that would happen.

Medicare & Medicaid

In 1968, Rep. Cecil King (D-CA), co-author with Sen. Clinton Anderson (D-NM) of legislation that evolved through often bitter debate into Medicare, was retiring from Congress. In the shadow of the Capitol building, down Independence Avenue, Health Education and Welfare Secretary Wilbur Cohen was conducting a ceremony in the department's North Building (since named the Wilbur Cohen building) to honor King.

Cohen enthusiastically told the assemblage of Washington health lobbyists, writers and staff members that "Cecil King had more to do with the passage of Medicare than any other person." King leapt to his feet. Wilbur," he began, "you and I know who had more to do with the passage of Medicare than any other person - Barry Goldwater." The audience burst into laughter. This story, when told inside the Beltway, never fails to get an appreciative response. Even outside the Beltway, it is a known political fact that Medicare, after years of controversy over any kind of national health financing program, was made possible by President Lyndon Baines Johnson's sweeping 1964 election victory over Sen. Barry Goldwater (R-Ariz.). Johnson, the consummate politician as Senate majority leader, vice president and the president, after John Kennedy's death, made skilled use of his landslide victory and the huge Senate and House majorities that rode into office on his coattails.

President Kennedy once said "politics is like football. If you see a hole in the line, go through it." Johnson did just that. Although many previous attempts had been fatally riddled by negative forces, Johnson overrode bitter opposition by the AMA, commercial insurers and political conservatives to make the long-sought dream of financing a health program for the elderly—and the needy, too—an historic possibility. With the help of Cohen and many others Johnson won an acceptable bill. He signed it in Independence, Mo., with Harry Truman at his side, grinning his approval. Here were two truly dedicated men who cast long standing opposition aside and won the landmark U.S. health care finance program.

By the time John F. Kennedy was elected president in 1960 it was clear the Social Security law would be the vehicle to carry Medicare health insurance for the elderly—just as FDR had considered doing. Social Security was, as AMA had feared, clearly a foot in the door for broader social programs.

Shortly before Kennedy took office, Rep. Aime Forand, (D-RI) had introduced a bill to provide health care for Social Security beneficiaries. The measure, which could not overcome conservative opposition, was re-introduced later. It lost a House Ways & Means Committee vote in 1960 but, despite the opposition, the snowball was gaining size and momentum. King and Anderson introduced a hospital insurance bill in 1961 with the support of the President. In May of 1962, Kennedy spoke to some 20,000 elderly people in New York's Madison Square Garden extolling the virtues of the legislation. Two days later AMA president Dr. Edward Annis attacked the Medicare proposal in a nationwide ratio address delivered (possibly to tweak Kennedy) from the same platform.

A bitter Congressional battle over Medicare continued through 1961 and 1962. AMA's American Medical Political Action Committee (AMPAC) representatives swarmed over Capitol Hill like an invading army, hoping to shoot down the hated legislation; operatives, meanwhile, worked the states during the Congressional election campaigns trying to get Republicans and/or conservatives elected. The Democrats managed to survive the elections but in the House, particularly, the margins were less than majestic. New York Sen. Jacob Javits, a moderate Republican, tried to find compromises that would blunt the opposition of the health industry, but his efforts were unsuccessful.

Then, tragically, the Ways & Means Committee hearings on the measure were interrupted by the Kennedy assassination. President Johnson moved swiftly to take political advantage of the national sorrow to win support for the Kennedy programs. In February 1964, he sent a special "Health of the Nation" message to Congress calling for immediate action on Medicare. But Medicare faced the test of the bitter 1964 presidential election. During the campaign the King-Anderson bill came to a Senate vote. Significantly, Goldwater, the Republican presidential candidate, made a special trip to the Capitol from his Arizona campaign headquarters to vote against

Medicare. The bill passed the Senate 49-44, but its further progress was held up by the need for a conference with the House which had passed quite a different bill.

Johnson campaigned hard for Medicare in his bid for election while Goldwater followed the conservative script. In a nationally televised speech, Governor Ronald Reagan of California, co-chairman of Californians for Goldwater, said: "I think we are telling our senior citizens that no one in this country should be denied medical care because of a lack of funds. But I think we are against forcing all citizens, regardless of need, into a compulsory government program, especially when we have such examples, as announced last week when France admitted that their medicare program was now bankrupt." The reference was a typical conservative tactic of comparing apples and oranges.

Although Medicare was not the only major issue in the campaign Johnson hit it hard in his folksy fashion and won election by one of the biggest pluralities in American history. On his coattails he carried 38 additional seats for the House, adding up to a ponderous 295-140 margin, and two more seats for the Senate, resulting in a 66-34 majority in that body.

Obviously impressed, no less than liberal Chairman Wilbur Mills (D-Ark.) of the Ways & Means Committee said he could support a payroll tax to pay for Medicare, as one does for Social Security. The next January the King-Anderson bill was introduced in the

Senate as S.1 and in the house as H.R.1—a tellingly symbolic honor.

AMA said it would fight to the end, but recognizing the facts of life came up with a counter proposal relying on health insurance companies and the states. The bill was called Eldercare. (During the 1996 presidential campaign, Bob Dole, who had been a House member from Kansas in 1965, noted that he had voted for Eldercare, apparently expecting no one would notice that he had supported a rival to Medicare rather than the bill that passed.)

As the Ways & Means Committee was seeking a solution to the differences between its pending legislation and conservative AMA demands for a private plan, Republican Rep. John Byrnes of Wisconsin, a member of Ways & Means, introduced a bill to create a voluntary federally administered "private" plan. Mills and the Democrats seized on the move as an opportunity to develop Medicare's Plan B, which used a voluntary plan to pay doctor bills as Part A paid hospital expense.

In an eventual compromise between the original Democratic plan for a hospital insurance program and conservative demands for a private plan and for a state-federal plan, Mills fashioned a recipe for what he called his "three-layer cake": Part A hospital insurance run by the Social Security Administration, a Part B plan in which beneficiaries would voluntarily pay a premium for medical services, and Medicaid, a state-federal cooperative health plan for the low-income populations.

Following passage of Medicare and Medicaid, Johnson was visited in the oval office by a delegation of AMA officials. Having been briefed by Cohen on what the doctors would want, Johnson was ready. The AMA officials wanted the president's assurance that the new law would never be used to interfere with the private practice of medicine in the U.S. Johnson turned to Cohen, Social Security Commissioner Robert Ball, outgoing HEW Secretary Anthony Celebrezze and incoming Secretary John Gardner and in mock stentorian tones said: "I want you to administer this program so it doesn't interfere in any way with the practice of medicine." The record doesn't show whether the AMA delegation got the joke but Cohen and Ball later assured confidants *they* did.

Medicine and Medicare both have changed a lot since then and AMA's attitude has grown more constructive as leaders have realized that doctor members were getting paid now where often in the past they did not.

Catastrophic Catastrophe

Danny Rostenkowski, baronial chairman of the House Ways & Means Committee which is usually referred to in news stories as powerful because it must originate bills levying taxes, was taken back when a group of outraged senior citizens surrounded his car on a busy Chicago street in August of 1989. The "assault" climaxed with a 69-year-old woman pounding on the hood of the congressman's automobile as he tried to escape.

"Impeach him!" cries echoed from the group of seniors estimated by the Chicago Tribune as 50 in number. "Rotten-kowski!" some shouted. Finally he stopped the car, broke free and ran away.

The incident, barely noticed at the time, triggered a series of events that resulted in repeal of the Medicare Catastrophic Coverage Act, a year after its enactment. Politicians, increasingly aware that the law was overdue, look back on the furor as an invaluable lesson in how public attitudes affect health care financing legislation. The angry seniors, prodded by organizations with political and financial ambitions, were protesting the new law's financial impact on them. For the most part they did not fully understand the law's complicated tax financing. Agitators had led them to belief the surcharge would be more expensive than it actually was. A Rostenkowski spokesman later told the Chicago Tribune: "Ninety percent of the people there wouldn't have to pay any tax at all." In fact, the law was enacted to help save them from severe healthcare costs.

The situation had greater meaning for health policy leaders because the catastrophic law would have paid for outpatient prescription drugs. This brought the strong and well-financed opposition of the prescription drug industry, historically fearing any government control over prices. After enactment of Medicare in 1965, the obvious question became how to protect seniors from the high cost of any catastrophic illness.

Because of rapidly rising health care costs that were becoming exorbitant for seniors living on limited pensions and Social Security, Medicare covered far less than the total cost of a major illness such as heart trouble or cancer. The cost-sharing they were enduring was putting some onto Medicaid which paid part of the extra costs for low income beneficiaries. The high cost of prescription drugs was much of the burden and Medicare did not cover drugs. The new catastrophic illness law did.

Well aware of the problem left unsolved by the Medicare program he ushered into law, Sen. Russell Long (D-La.) began to look for ways to close the gap. In 1971 he proposed a catastrophic illness insurance plan which, along with a proposal to add the disabled to Medicare, amounted to what his aides called an interim national health insurance bill, in effect moving Medicare toward a national plan covering more than the aged.

He suggested the idea after hearing his House counterpart, Chairman Wilbur Mills (D-Ark.) of the

Ways & Means Committee, talk favorably about the idea of catastrophic illness insurance coverage. Long was joined by a prominent member of his Finance Committee, Sen. Abraham Ribicoff (D-Conn.). It became increasingly clear that those who had seen the need for Medicare saw the necessary next step to complement health care insurance for the aged.

Although Catastrophic never rose to the level of a serious legislative proposal the idea was becoming increasingly popular. Late in 1985 Otis R. Bowen, MD, Secretary of Health and Human Services, joined his dynamic special assistant Thomas R. Burke in writing an article for the FAH Review, a magazine published by the Federation of American Hospitals, an association of for-profit, or "investor-owned" hospitals, as they liked to call them. In the article the two men outlined a proposal "for restructuring the Medicare benefit package in a manner that will provide catastrophic acute inpatient and outpatient care to Medicare beneficiaries in a cost neutral manner."

The proposal, which grew out of a presidentially appointed committee investigating the status of Medicare chaired by Dr. Bowen, recognized that at that time 65 to 70 percent of Medicare beneficiaries were purchasing Medigap policies to cover co-pay deductibles of Medicare. Bowen sought to acquire comparable and often superior benefits at a fraction of the cost. Bowen and Burke calculated that catastrophic illness costs of a few Medicare recipients would be borne by an added premium to be paid by all 28 million beneficiaries.

The idea proved popular enough for President Reagan to include it in his 1987 State of the Union address. Reagan promised to "remove a financial spectre facing our older Americans—the fear of an illness so expensive that it can result in having to make an intolerable choice between bankruptcy and death...I will submit legislation shortly to help free the elderly from the fear of catastrophic illness."

Reagan and his advisers knew exactly what they were talking about. The cost of being sick was proving so increasingly expensive that even the heralded Medicare plan was inadequate to still the worries of less-than-wealthy older Americans.

Legislation sent to Congress by Reagan's Department of Health and Human Services proposed a Medicare Catastrophic Coverage Act. Since Reagan, who feared taxes more than the other inevitability, insisted that the expanded coverage be paid for by the beneficiaries themselves—like an insurance plan. The proposal called for a "supplemental premium" to be "folded into" the voluntary Part B medical insurance addition to Medicare. Any citizen over 65 was automatically eligible for free hospital insurance. Those who chose to, as most did, paid a premium for the Part B plan. What the catastrophic proposal did was insure costs above usual Medicare payments, which were limited to restrain certain cost inflation. Many elders who could afford it had been insuring themselves against catastrophic costs by paying for Medicap.

Bowen originally proposed a $5 a month additional cost to pay for the new benefits. But as the legislation moved through Rostenkowski's Ways & Means Committee, the Senate Finance Committee and the office of Sen. Lloyd Bentsen (D-Tex.), the potential costs—with such additions as a prescription drug benefit—began to grow faster than payment estimates. There was no question that the biggest cost hazard that seniors faced under Medicare was the mounting cost of medication which was not covered by Medicare.

At times when controversial legislation is making its way toward law, Washington is like a jungle with high-paid lobbyists for many different causes or financial interests lurking behind every column. These legendary big spenders are on the lookout for something that might irk their clients so they can prove how valuable they are. At the same time professional societies are eager to show their dues-paying members how important membership in their societies can be. When the prescription drug industry sees a threat to its profits, lobbyists are turned loose. In the case of catastrophic health insurance the threat perceived by drug manufacturers was the strong possibility federal regulation could control drug prices once the government started paying prescription drug costs for many millions of people.

Drug industry lobbyists worked hard, as Washington lobbyists can do—if one categorizes expense account lunches and dinner as work—in a bitter effort to keep a drug benefit out of Medicare Catastrophic. The industry's fear of government controls evidently overwhelmed any interest in potential added profits. Heavy lobbying was set in motion by the Pharmaceutical Manufacturers Association and by individual manufacturers. The intense interest in stopping a drug benefit for the nation's elderly was remarkable in the light of a Congressional Budget Office estimate that the catastrophic health cost benefit would pay for more than $5 billion worth of drugs during the first five years. The Department of HHS set the potential cost higher, more than $3 billion the first year alone.

Despite the lobbying by drug interests and others the law was passed overwhelmingly by Congress in June of 1988 to be signed in the White House rose garden by a triumphant President Reagan.

But the fast-emerging difficulties in getting the law through Congress amounted to a gathering storm that would eventually prove fatal. Organizations vying for elderly members were already seeking to show that the government had rendered more of a disservice than a service and that they would address the basically fictional grievances if enough dues were paid.

Actually, the administration didn't help the new law when the Internal Revenue Service printed new 1989 tax forms with reminders that the added premium would have to be paid along with due taxes by seniors covered by Medicare Part B. The amounts were determined by the new law based on the taxpayer's income. Despite Regan's insistence that the benefit be self-financing, its appearance on a tax form have it every appearance of a tax.

One of the many senior groups that jumped at the opportunity to attract new dues-paying members had been organized, ironically, by James Roosevelt, one of the sons of President Franklin D. Roosevelt who created the Social Security law to which Medicare had been appended as additional titles. James Roosevelt had already used his National Committee to Preserve Social Security and Medicare to win new friends by addressing the problem of Social Security "notch babies"—people ineligible for the program's cash benefits because they were born before Social Security benefits took effect.

Roosevelt immediately set in motion a publicity campaign of the sort used to sell items to the unsuspecting. He mailed extravagantly worded broadsides informing seniors that "rich and powerful special interest groups are wielding more power in Washington than ever before." The huge direct mail campaign said that for a mere $10 investment the recipient would have the protection of Roosevelt's committee against "those in Congress and the administration who want to unfairly change these successful programs in order to give tax cuts or subsidies to wealthy and powerful special interests." The law, he said, would require "millions of seniors to pay an income tax surcharge of up to $1,600 per couple ($800 for singles)." In reality couples with incomes over $70,000 would pay the $1,600 maximum.

The well-managed outcry of many similarly opportunistic groups rose to such a pitch that members of Congress were unable and unwilling to ignore them. Both the White House and Congress were bombarded by so many complaints that it was only a matter of time before the Catastrophic law was repealed in 1989. Every thought of trying to restore the benefits with less offensive financing was instantly lost to political realities. President George Bush, who had been elected before the repeal took place, never showed any interest in reviving the dream of his predecessor.

The lesson for successors who envision restoring the dream of drugs under Medicare was indelible.

HMO and Managed Care

History can be made quietly in obscure places. A sea change in the American medical care system occurred at a historical meeting February 5, 1970, in a room of the unpretentious DuPont Plaza hotel on Washington's Connecticut Avenue rented by Dr. Paul Ellwood of the American Rehabilitation Foundation in Minneapolis. HMOs were born here.

They were fathered by the federal government and the private medical sector. Whether it was a noble birth or a mismatch producing a monster was and is today a subject of strong opinions in many places. The meeting was the result of an inquiry by Nixon Administration Department of Health, Education and Welfare Undersecretary John (Jack) Veneman. The group christened prepaid group practices "Health Maintenance Organizations" and started a movement that was to rise to near dominance of American medical care financing.

The idea was not new but the energetic Ellwood, who was later to rename his think tank Interstudy, had been contemplating how to use it on a large scale to save money. Early in the 20th century the Mayo brothers, a pair of Rochester, MN physicians, founded a non-profit clinic. Called a group practice, it was not prepaid in the form of insurance and never has been. But the idea of group practices was beginning to flower. About the same time, two Los Angeles, CA, doctors, Donald Ross and H. Clifford Loos, began contracting to provide medical care for city employees and their dependants. In Palo Alto, CA, a colorful Stanford Medical School graduate, Dr. Russel Lee, put together a group practice in defiance of American Medical Association leaders who were showing increasing opposition to the idea of doctors working on salary.

Another California physician, Dr. Sidney Garfield, established a group practice under contract to care for construction workers building the Los Angeles Auqueduct in California's Mojave Desert. His innovation attracted the attention of industrialist Henry J. Kaiser and his son Edgar. They organized the Kaiser Permanente (Permanente being the name of a nearby river) Medical Care Program for construction workers building Grand Coulee Dam in Washington State.

World War II was the next step for Kaiser Permanente, as it was for other economic sectors. The plan provided medical care for workers at Kaiser shipyards building "victory ships" in the San Francisco and Vancouver, WA, regions. The idea was so popular with workers that it became a community-wide facility. But progress is never easy and the opposition of AMA to this conceived threat to fee-for-service medicine inflamed a battle threatening to rival the war that had just ended.

AMA represented the majority, but not all, of the nation's physicians. For the most part the opposition came from more conservative members and paid staff who magnified opposition to group practice to stay in good favor with the conservative leadership. AMA had opposed the idea of medical practice becoming anything other than independent physicians working without interference from government. The opposition was based on a combination of professional pride and the desire to make lots of money.

The idea, clearly one whose time had come, was developed in the District of Columbia, where the Group Health Association was founded, and in New York which saw the opening of Health Insurance Plan, both of which have continued to operate as major plans.

Ellwood, Veneman, HEW health policy experts Tom Joe—a colorful blind Korean—and Lewis Butler and several others discussed the idea of prepaid group practices being used to help reduce the government's rising contributions to the new programs Medicare and Medicaid. The Nixon administration officials were lured by the prospect for savings in a fast-rising governmental cost area. As too often became the case, it was costs, not quality of care, that stimulated the passion for change. This not to say no one cared about the patients' welfare, but money was the driving force.

Veneman and the others saw great possibilities for the Administration and the group decided to call the new payment form Health Maintenance Organizations to emphasize the role of preventive health measures. Since Medicare had grown to be a much bigger government cost than expected, it was decided to propose to Congress a new Medicare Part C which could pay the costs of Part A hospital insurance and Part B medical costs for any beneficiary who chose this over customary separate payments.

The idea was offered to Congress by Nixon's HEW and, after a back yard barbecue conference between Veneman and House Ways & Means Chairman Wilbur Mills (D-Ark.)—who could be real folksy—the committee approved the new wrinkle. The proposal made it through Mills's committee but was held captive in the Senate Finance Committee, where staff opposition proved fatal.

Finance Committee health aide Jay Constantine, a scrappy liberal who adopted the role of watchdog over unnecessary expenses, immediately objected to what he saw as the possibility of HMOs being money machines rather than simply healthcare organizations. He saw the Part C proposal as a "blank check" through which entrepreneurs could get rich from what was designed as a social program. His opposition was forward-looking and prophetic. HMOs have through the years become increasingly for-profit. But the idea of moving Medicare patients into HMOs—which had been promoted by the Nixon administration—was moved to the back shelf and did not happen until a decade later, during the George H.W. Bush administration. Nixon liked the HMO idea and approved plans developed by his aides that resulted in a big government program to stimulate HMO development.

The fact is, the meeting in Ellwood's room was the beginning of the largest change in the American health care financing system. In was a signal event that changed the thrust of medical care financing from simple insurance financing of doctor or hospital-patient relationships to the system of group medicine that AMA had traditionally feared.

The next step after Nixon discovered HMOs and stimulated their growth came in March of 1983 when the Robert Wood Johnson Foundation and the National Governors' Association announced a $9.6 million grant program to look into expansions of the HMO idea. The title of the effort was "Program for Prepaid Managed Health Care," the first mention of the now universal term Managed Care that can be found in the health policy archives.

To come were variations on the theme such as Preferred Provider Organization in which a plan member could use any doctor wanted from a list of the "preferred providers" the financing group suggested, or go out of network at a higher cost. The variations continued to grow as managers sought to meet the complaints of occasional patients that they couldn't get the treatment they wanted in the way they wanted it.

In an odd twist, even as President Nixon sought to make use of the prepaid group practice idea, his eventual successor, then California Gov. Ronald Reagan, was trying to save Medicaid money by encouraging eligibles to join Prepaid Health Plans. But the quickly organized movement was courting unfavorable headlines with such promotion gimmicks as free chicken dinners; and it soon collapsed.

As the prepaid groups practice method grew and expanded, patients who found it less than ideal began to complain more and more. They couldn't get the attention they wanted, or the medications, or the tests.

They were encountering lines and waiting lists for treatments. Most complaints arose from limitations on tests, drugs, surgical procedures and the like.

And physicians who couldn't deliver care the way they wanted—restrictions on tests being an example—also began to complain or to seek subsidies.

It goes without saying that economies cannot be reached nor costs cut without cutting back on some expenses. And in order to make the managed care omelette, providers and insurers were breaking a lot of eggs.

A young physician, Dr. Michael Brazda, loaded with idealism to heal the sick and new to practice, said with a measure of frustration, "I read the New England Journal of Medicine every week and study 'the case of the week.' But they go wild on tests, and I cannot give anywhere near the tests I want to help the patient because the plan won't let me. All they ever talk about is costs."

To be sure the restrictions didn't come out of whole cloth. There had been abuses. Many tests charged to the patients' insurers are unnecessary. Too often the overtesting is related to physician ownership of the labs. And much of it is pure defensive medicine in an increasingly desperate effort by providers to avoid often unethical malpractice suits.

Jackson Hole

In the late 1970s, Health, Education and Welfare Secretary Joseph Califano, former aide to President Lyndon B. Johnson, contacted Stanford University economics professor Alain Enthoven to ask his help in a project for President Jimmy Carter. Carter was expecting a challenge for the Democratic presidential nomination in 1980 from Sen. Edward M. Kennedy (D-Mass.) who was still offering a national health plan as one of his campaign platform planks. Califano was looking for a better health care idea to use in beating off Kennedy's challenge. Enthoven had concluded that there was only one path to the national health care goal searched for by so many for so long to such great disappointment: open market economic competition.

"I had in mind that competition would naturally lead away from traditional indemnity insurance toward capitated plans," he later said. He referred to the prepaid group model where a single pre-payment per individual covers whatever the policy allows, known formally as capitation—and as rationing to detractors.

Carter beat down Kennedy's dramatic challenge at the Democratic national convention in New York's Madison Square Garden but was defeated in the general election by the popular conservative Republican icon Ronald Reagan, former movie star and California governor.

Enthoven continued his pursuit of an answer nevertheless. In special articles published in two 1989 issues of the New England Journal of Medicine, Enthoven and his partner Richard Kronick proposed that "everyone not covered by Medicare, Medicaid or some other public program be enabled to buy affordable coverage" either through their employers or through a "public sponsor" such as the U.S. government.

Enthoven had for several years been promoting his plan which he called "Consumer Choice Health Plan." Essential to his proposal was what he came to call "managed competition," in which purchasers of health plans would stimulate competition between insurers for business. The proposal addressed a widespread national situation in which many businesses bought insurance for their employees as a benefit. Enthoven's plan would "mandate" that businesses do just that.

The competition, long favored by conservatives as an alternative to government health insurance, would call for "intelligent collective agents, called sponsors, to contract with competing health plans and continuously monitor and adjust the market to overcome its tendencies to failure," Enthoven said. The key idea was that sponsors would manage the "process of informed, cost-conscious consumer choice that would offer the reward of more subscribers to health plans whose providers delivered high-quality care economically."

His words were tempting to the thriving business of health: operate by the dictates of the market and the business of health will continue to be healthy whether or not the uninsured will be. But about that time, in the late 1980s, those health insurers began to take note of the fact that liberal designs on a government solution were continuing and that escalating medical care costs were directing the attention of businesses who paid the bills to the national health care program across the border in Canada as a possible model of "single payer" insurance, the payer being the government. The numbers of uninsured were growing in an age that saw increasing technology and an oversupply of health care providers. This situation was particularly difficult for those not solvent or eligible for government health programs. Commercial insurers were very worried, particularly the smaller insurers that had banded together in the Health Insurance Association of America (HIAA). They feared that larger insurers and HMOs would damage their business. Also concerned were some of the nonprofit insurers such as Blue Cross and Blue Shield and Kaiser Permanente.

Then the scene shifts back to Dr. Paul Ellwood of HMO fame. Father of the name HMO if not the idea itself, Ellwood had conducted a 25-year search for an answer to the nation's health care financing needs. Meanwhile, it so happens, he had invested large amounts of money in a resort facility at Jackson Hole, Wyo., where the Union Pacific had many years before built a resort to encourage train travel. Ellwood, Enthoven and several others had been meeting regularly at Jackson Hole to discuss national health care financing problems in a context revolving around Enthoven's managed competition model. In February of 1990 Ellwood and Enthoven joined with a group of health insurers in the first of a series of expanded meetings at Ellwood's Jackson Hole condo. Their work attracted such national figures as Bernard (Barney) Tresnowski of Blue Cross, William Link of Prudential, Dr. David Lawrence of Kaiser Permanente, Thomas Pyle of the Harvard Community health plan, and others.

Tresnowski was one of the prime movers. He called a highly experienced health care policy analyst, Lynn Etheredge, who had served four administrations in the Office of Management and Budget, and asked him to help found a meeting group. The insurers were the principal financial backers of the historical meeting. But remarkably the discussions did not revolve necessarily around the needs of the uninsured, nor even politics with an election coming, but around the business of health. It was a business meeting. The Blues were nonprofit at the time but many proved to be on the way toward going commercial. Kaiser has always been nonprofit and has stayed that way, but wanted to have a look anyway. Lawrence had gotten the impression that the Jackson Hole Group (JHG) might have an influence on national policy. Before the realities began to dawn on them, many of the commercial insurers had at times been heard referring to Enthoven and Ellwood as enemies who were out to push for a national program replacing the insurance industry. The apparent aim of the insurers was to find a national plan that would, through competition, more or less reduce costs by forcing a marketing plan that would appeal to larger insurers. An outbreak of mergers of commercial and nonprofit health insurers and hospitals was getting underway.

Representatives of American Medical Association and the hospital industry were there to watch. The group, which had already been dubbed the JHG by reporters who saw a story developing, began meeting frequently. Health insurance companies were generous in their provision of the cost that Ellwood needed to keep his mountain lair healthy.

The insurers recognized that traditional health insurance in the U.S., both for and not for profit, was going to have to change and managed care was fast emerging as the way to go. The initial point at least was to keep the government as far away as possible so the insurers could continue to do business.

Later that year, 1991, an alarm bell went off that electrified all parties, particularly the JHG and workers in the Bill Clinton presidential campaign who had been watching JGH closely. It was set off by the tragic death of Republican Sen. John Heinz of Pennsylvania, who was killed in a plane crash. Harris Wofford, a colorful liberal Democrat, was appointed to Heinz's seat in the U.S. Senate and won a special election allowing him to complete the term. Wofford, a tireless civil rights advocate in the South, had nudged history many years earlier when he persuaded Sen. John F. Kennedy (D-Mass.) to call Coretta King, wife of the Rev. Martin Luther King Jr., and express his sympathy over King's arrest in Atlanta on a trumped-up traffic charge. Historians believe the liberal support that Kennedy won with this public act was instrumental in helping him to win the presidential nomination back in 1960.

Wofford won Heinz's seat in a special election against Republican Dick Thornburgh, a former two-term governor of Pennsylvania and aide to President Nixon who was favored to win the election. Wofford seized on an issue that he believed was ready for public attention—health. He called for national health insurance. Thornburgh opposed the idea.

Wofford's upset victory was instantly interpreted as a sign that health had arrived as an issue. Ironically, Wofford lost the next election in 1994 to Rick Santorum, who was strongly supported by the National Rifle Association.

Presidential candidates vying for the Democratic nomination (in 1991) to oppose President George Bush had lined up with proposals for national health care plans in hand. Sen. Bob Kerrey (D-NE) proposed a universal health care plan financed by earmarked taxes. Arkansas Gov. Bill Clinton called for universal health care coverage paid for by savings from government-imposed cost controls and reduction of billing fraud and abuse.

The next year the JHG issued "A Proposal for Reform" that said The Jackson Hole Concept was a competitive health system where health insurance and health care competition is motivated, structured and regulated to reward with the *most customers* those health organizations who get the best health results at the lowest costs." The proposal went on to call for delivery of health care through Accountable Health Partnerships, "managed care-like organizations that are publicly accountable for their health outcomes." Then, the plan added, small employers would purchase coverage from competing Health Insurance Purchasing Cooperatives (HPICs) which would arrange for consumers to get coverage from competing AHPs. It was the answer that most of the group wanted: let the business of health go on as a business. Just give it another name. Hopes for a true universal health insurance plan were dashed again by financial and political opposition.

The Clinton Fiasco

Governor Bill Clinton of Arkansas wanted to be president of the United States. In developing a strategy to secure the Democratic nomination with the assistance of a legion of advisers, Clinton became acutely aware of what a telling issue healthcare coverage could be.

And, as governor of a state with a large number of low income citizens, he got a first- hand look through Medicaid at the fast-growing problem of hospital costs. He was alarmed and wanted to do something about it for the good of the nation. Clinton assembled a group of advisers, many of whom were eventually to join his White House staff. One of these was Ira Magaziner, an old friend whom he had gotten to know when both men were Rhodes Scholars at Oxford.

Magaziner had gone on from his scholarship days to become a one man think tank. At Brown University he became famous for a painstaking study of the curriculum which eventually resulted in a new age revision of the way the ivy-covered school taught. He then moved company by company into doing the same for industry in his own intensive strategic planning style. Magaziner attempted to tell General Electric how to make better refrigerators and Wang how to improve computers, as both companies neared bankruptcy. His experience in the health field was confined to time and motion studies for hospitals.

Clinton asked Magaziner to help him develop the health policy that he thought would be vital to his campaign for the Democratic nomination and the Presidency. Magaziner contacted Walter Zelman, who had worked with California Insurance Commissioner John Garamendi in a quest for "global" budgeting in which payments for health care would be designed to cover the patient's entire medical experience, from tongue depressor to hospital discharge.

Magaziner also signed up Paul Starr, Princeton University health economist and author; Brice Fried, California health policy expert, and a Harvard medical student, Atul Gawandi, among others. They had been watching the Jackson Hole Group and brought in Enthoven & Co. Managed Competition seemed to fit right in with what they were looking for: a silver bullet for the Clinton campaign health plank that would risk no danger of being called socialized medicine.

It was enough to convince the Democratic primary voters, and Gov. Clinton was nominated for president with Sen. Albert Gore of Tennessee as his vice-presidential running mate. Although Gore had become associated with health policy often as a U.S. Senator, he was more or less distant from the exercise that was to come. As Clinton jumped into the fray, President George H.W. Bush countered with an elaborate plan devised by his health advisers, led by Health Care Financing Administration (HCFA) chief Gail Wilensky. The Bush plan embraced competition and managed care to satisfy conservatives. It encouraged small employers to buy insurance for their workers through purchasing cooperatives. But national health care financing, and the likely inclusion of taxes, was such a tender subject it was initially ignored.

Gov. Clinton outlined the plan his advisers had been talking about in a September 24, 1991 speech at the Merck Pharmaceutical plant in Rahway, NJ. He pledged that within the first 100 days of a Clinton Administration he would submit "a comprehensive health care plan for real change that deals with costs and coverage and access, with quality and the maintenance of consumer choice." He said he would require employers to cover their employees while the government covered the unemployed in a program which would require people "to pay in accordance with their ability to pay and not more." Generally he outlined a program not dissimilar from the Jackson Hole proposal and said his forthcoming plan would not require new taxes and was not "play or pay," a system whereby employers must insure their workers or pay into a fund to insure the uninsured.

In a campaign document—the paperback book "Putting People First"—Clinton and Gore declared that instead of putting people first, Washington had favored the insurance companies, drug manufacturers and health-care bureaucracies. "We cannot build tomorrow's economy until we guarantee every American the right to affordable quality health care," they said.

Their book promised national spending caps, universal coverage, managed care networks and elimination of drug price gouging. They also vowed to take on the insurance industry, fight bureaucracy and billing fraud, and provide a rational medical liability system, a core benefits package and equitable costs. In other words, just about every idea that sounded good at that time.

The plan to deliver this heaven on earth campaign promise did not exist in any detail, but the effort to find it was to come.

In a televised campaign debate with President Bush, Clinton said if some states and other countries can provide health care plans "American can do it, too. I'm tired of being told we can't. I say we can. We can do better, and we must."

After Gov. Clinton was elected president, he assigned his wife, Hillary Rodham Clinton, and Ira Magaziner to the task of developing the all-encompassing health care program he had promised. Mrs. Clinton, an experienced lawyer, was a newcomer to the health field as was Magaziner.

With his background as a corporate organizer, Magaziner set out to overhaul the nation's health care system as he had done as a consultant to major manufacturers. He announced plans to appoint a committee of 500 to study the problem of how the president could in 100 days set in motion the wheels to solve an historic problem—a move that was to haunt him later as conservatives began to learn the identity of liberal members.

At the same time, President Clinton was organizing the rest of his government and made what was probably one of his worst decisions as far as his health care program was concerned. He persuaded Sen. Lloyd Bentsen (D-Tex.) To leave the Senate and become his Secretary of the Treasury. With this appointment he removed from the Senate the chairman of the powerful Finance Committee, which would be vastly important in processing whatever legislative remedy the Administration was to send to Congress. Bentsen, who had dealt with health financing legislation for years, was dedicated and considerably knowledgeable about the subject.

To make matters worse, Bentsen's removal from the Finance Committee automatically moved Sen. Daniel Patrick (Pat) Moynihan (D-NY), a veteran politician but an erratic (some called him "colorful") intellectual, to the chairmanship. Moynihan, who had worked for President Nixon as a White House staffer, was apparently undergoing a political change of life that eventually saw the New York liberal talk seriously about "privatizing" Social Security, one of the nation's most experienced and revered social programs begun by FDR.

Then Magaziner began his strategic planning attempt to, in the words of one disenchanted staffer, "reinvent the wheel." Rather than examine the health care situation through the eyes of experienced individuals who had been working on it for years; Magaziner appointed to his committee of 500 many members who were inexperienced in health policy. And they often met in secret. Among the many available experts who were kept away from the talks was Secretary Bentsen, who later said that he sometimes learned of events from the newspapers as committee members began to systematically leak details of the deliberations to chosen reporters.

Bentsen appeared to regard Magaziner as some sort of staff person. At one point he heard that Magaziner, the so-called "health czar," had gone to Capitol Hill to meet with legislative leaders he had never met before and had greeted them with: "Hello fellas. Let's get to work."

Subcommittees of the Committee of 500 began to discuss a health program somewhere in between the Jackson Hole plan and the Garamendi California plan brought in to the discussions by Starr, the Princeton economist, and Zelman, the former Garamendi lieutenant. But increasingly bitter opposition to the proposed plan grew among natural enemies as stories leaked to the press told of cutting Medicare and Medicaid to pay for the plan—horrifying hospitals which depended heavily on the programs. Opposition came as well from the commercial health insurance industry which saw a threat to the economic futures of investors and from small business organizations that saw the unwelcome threat of regulation and mandates to insure workers.

Employer mandates were unpopular from the beginning with conservatives and small business. They were perhaps a birth defect that turned fatal. Congressional concerns with passing any new taxes were another burden that proved too heavy for the package.

As talk of a network of regulatory boards such as Jackson Hole and Garamendi had envisioned was reported, Moynihan told a public television program he regarded it as "fantasy." His critique proved to be insightful but was not what the president needed.

In September of 1993 President Clinton appeared before a joint session of Congress and a national television audience to announce that his wife and her group had achieved a "Health Security" plan that would replace the flood of paperwork then necessary to file health claims with insurance companies with "one standard insurance form." Veteran Washington hands thought it ironic that he named the proposal what Sen. Edward Kennedy (D-Mass.) had called his "controversial organized labor-backed NHI plan" two decades before. Clinton foresaw a comprehensive national plan that would improve the quality of care and do it cheaper through a complex system that had only begun to be shown through the usual charts and alphabet titles.

The Congress was led by Democrats, but immediately, thanks to advanced stories, it became highly critical of the innovative and complex proposal. Rep. Fortney (Pete) Stark (D-CA), who was later to propose an alternative Medicare-for-All plan, said the President showed that "managed competition is to health care what the Laffer curve was to economics—a hope and a prayer and an untested theory." The independent-minded Congressional Budget Office said that the savings from Medicare and Medicaid and other spending cuts, as well as savings from fraud and abuse control, could not produce the money needed to implement the President's plan, deflating the politically motivated no-tax, easy-out proposal.

The usual professional, vested and political interests opposing government involvement began to unload their heavy artillery. One of the most novel negative campaigns came from the Health Insurance Association of America which blanketed the country with radio commercials featuring a mythical couple, Harry and Louise, who complained of the damage the Clinton bill would do to their lives. What really concerned the HIAA was the damage the bill would do to the association's members.

The road was rough before the president and his people began to journey down it. Then the potholes grew to canyon-like proportions. In a move to please both sides, Tennessee Democratic Congressman James Cooper, who called himself a conservative Democrat, jumped into the battle with his own bill. He called it "Clinton lite," but his bill only asked that employers make health insurance available to their employees—hardly a politically dangerous idea. His bill paid no attention to the poor who couldn't afford insurance. The conservatives liked it, as could be expected, and it took votes from the Clinton bill.

Senate Democratic leader George Mitchell (Me.) and House Democratic leader Dick Gephardt (Mo.) each put in their own versions of the Clinton bill, which were crafted to look like the original but with compromises that might help them squeeze by. There were key differences. Clinton's bill relied on a mandate that employers pay 80 percent of the costs of employee health plans, and the Gephardt bill was similar in its financing. But Mitchell called for increasing the tobacco tax and the tax on handgun ammunition along with an added tax on health insurance premiums to pay for the uninsured.

Mitchell, who was once chairman of the Senate Finance Committee's Health Subcommittee, was out to lunch on this one. He later retired from the Senate and joined a Washington law firm that represented tobacco interests among others. Clinton's impossible dream needed a Senate leader and Mitchell was not it.

When the major committees of Congress finally took up the bill, in May of 1994, leading members had prepared an arsenal of amendments to address problems that had appeared as opponents leveled their guns at Hillary's and Ira's product.

Much of the opposition in Congress was led by Sen. Bob Dole (Kans.), Republican majority leader who was winding up for a campaign to oppose Clinton in the 1996 election. The twist by Dole was ironic. A long-time supporter of health legislation, he had often pointed to the need for a national health plan that was dramatized when he returned from World War II, badly wounded, and in need of medical treatment beyond what the Veterans Hospitals offered. Dole would tell of people in his home town of Russell, Kansas, handing around cigar boxes to collect funds to help send him to a hospital in Chicago. He had worked with Sen. Russell Long to get health legislation through the

Finance Committee and was regarded by Long as a willing and helpful partner.

But the Clinton bill and leadership proposals prompted Dole to utter the political cliches as old as the conservative movement: the bills, he said, "prescribe more government, more taxes and more entitlements." Dole was pandering to conservatives in his ambition to succeed Clinton and the dread thought of Clinton signing a national health bill when Dole was running for his own Rose Garden privileges was too much for the dour Kansan who was a leading opponent of any version of the measure, compromises included.

As the legislation appeared more clearly to be stranded, one of the most respected men in the Senate, John Chafee, a Republican from Rhode Island, sought to save the day for the American people with a proposed bi-partisan compromise, but he suffered abuse from his own party for his efforts. Former aides to Chafee and the Finance Committee tell of hearing committee conservatives shouting abuse at Chafee behind closed doors. At one point the Congressman told his staff that rather than suffer the abuse he had seen and felt, he would refrain from ever sponsoring health care legislation again. Happily, in successive years, he abandoned that resolve and became active again on health legislation. During a 1998 inter-party battle on patient protection legislation Chafee again sought to help forge compromises.

Conservatives were not the only opponents the Clinton bill met in Congress. Sen. Bob Kerrey (D-NE), one of the group of senators working with Chafee on a compromise and himself a presidential aspirant, came out in opposition to the White House proposal in what became a growing Kerrey campaign against any sort of entitlement program, including Social Security. The American Medical Association flirted briefly with the Clinton plan early in the game, but when Congressional Republicans objected, AMA pulled back and never endorsed the Administration bill.

Despite strong attempts by the President, Mrs. Clinton and their aides, the nation's uninsured were left begging. Poor handling, the secret planning sessions, the failure to make use of existing knowledge in a fumbling attempt to reinvent the wheel, and the bitter opposition of commercial, political and professional self interests—all had combined to deal the fatal blows to a national health care plan whose time should have come.

The Collapse

Arnold S. Relman, M.D., scholarly editor of the prestigious New England Journal of Medicine (known in the medical profession as NEJM), startled the medical world on October 23, 1980 when he featured a special article which he had written himself. Relman opened by noting that President Dwight D. Eisenhower, in his farewell address on January 17, 1961, had warned his countrymen of what he called the "military-industrial complex." The President, Relman noted, "was concerned about the possible conflict between public and private interests in the crucial area of national defense."

Taking a page from the President and former five-star general, Relman warned of a "new medical-industrial complex…a large and growing network of private corporations engaged in the business of supplying healthcare services to patients for profit—services heretofore provided by nonprofit institutions or individual practitioners." This he saw as "an unprecedented phenomenon with broad and potentially troubling implications for the future of our medical care system."

It took a while before the healthcare world began to realize the implications of what Relman had said, but he was, indeed, a voice crying in the wilderness. Relman was not the only person to see storm clouds building in the form of for-profit hospitals and managed care companies, but he was a brave and bold prophet. What he saw and pointed to was the developing invasion of for-profit medical management that was eventually to collapse in a heap with several for-profit hospital administrators being sent to jail for fraud and for-profit HMOs losing their grip on the public and professional management to the point where HMO jokes got laughs in movies. Resulting cries of protest would raise serious government and private questions about the suitability of HMOs as Medicare contractors.

Relman raised the question that has dominated discussions of the subject since: Who is the intended beneficiary of all this, the patient or the investor? This question has dominated the discussion since Relman's historic "special article" and likely will remain center stage in the debate between conservatives who believe business is sacred and thus the investor is the concern, and moderate-to-liberal observers who say the patient comes first and quality is the goal. At an expensive reception hosted by a provider group, a cynical guest who was asked to offer a toast raised his glass to "the wonderful people who made all this possible—the sick."

Relman, the physician-editor, noted early that "proprietary hospitals are not new in this country." Many small hospitals and clinics have been founded by physicians, as were group practices. But their aim was better, more affordable medical care, not fat profits.

In the mid-1960s, administrators and stockholders of for-profit hospitals concluded that American Hospital Association, the blanket national association of hospitals, was, in the words of an observer, "not fighting for return on equity" for profit-making hospitals. AHA was dominated by voluntary, not-for-profit hospitals which wanted profits only to finance capital equipment and charity care, not return on investments. Members of the citizens board of Providence Hospital in the District of Columbia heard talk by the Daughters of Charity, the nuns who run the hospital, about "profits." But they needed money for what an observer at AHA called their "rainy day" fund. The institutions require a bank account to finance needs "all over the board," he said.

Hospitals have seen an increasing flood of uninsured patients over the years. Many go into the emergency rooms like the insured go to their doctors' offices. In one survey hospitals reported five to eight percent of their patients were uninsured. The number has continued to rise, becoming a continuing national problem.

In 1999, the New England Journal of Medicine itself quoted a Dartmouth Medical School report showing that investor-owned hospitals are charging Medicare more per beneficiary than nonprofits. The figures were quite accusatory.

It never takes long before the realities prompt common interests, like for-profit hospitals, to form national organizations to represent their more narrow views before the federal government, both the executive branch and Congress. The Federation of American Hospitals was formed in 1966 to represent commercial, or investor-owned hospitals, as they preferred to be called after public relations advisors suggested a less graphic name.

The for-profit hospital industry rose to the heights and fell to the depths in the public estimation through a series of purchases and mergers that began in 1987 when a smart and ambitious young executive, Richard Scott, created the Columbia Hospital Corporation and began accumulating more institutions. By 1994, Columbia Hospital Corporation had absorbed more than 150 institutions through a merger with Hospital Corporation of America. The resultant Columbia/HCA was worth $25 billion by 1997. It was growing so fast that one cynical observer said it was "socialism in reverse." Rather than the government taking over as conservatives warned, big business was the dominant player. Doctors and patients began complaining that the drive for profits was demeaning quality of care.

Then the relentless quest for profits from illness exploded. In March of 1997 agents of the FBI, IRS, US Attorney's office, the Departments of Health and Human Services and the Defense Department raided Columbia/HCA's offices in El Paso, TX, where Scott started out, and carried out huge boxes of files.

The agents were looking for evidence of Medicare and Medicaid fraud. Four executives of Columbia/HCA were indicted. Numerous executives were fired by Thomas Frist Jr., who became head executive upon the resignation under fire of Scott. Frist is a brother of Sen. Bill Frist (R-TN). The senator is a heart surgeon who held stock in the corporation started by their father, Thomas Frist Sr. The Congressional Ethics Office said later it was permissible for Frist to vote on controversial healthcare legislation even if he had such investments.

Scott's grandiose dream of transforming the majority of the nation's hospitals into one- stop health centers, which he had so breathlessly described to investment analysts, had collapsed. Money, rather than the welfare of patients, had become the principal object, and when this happens the most greedy of human traits can take over.

"Columbia hospitals exist to make money—period." Eric Gardner, manager of three Columbia hospitals, made the statement in an explosive story in the May 30, 1997 issue of The Wall Street Journal. Gardner said he was eager to testify at the trial of Columbia/HCA executives. Managers were, he said, graded on report cards on how well they were performing in making money for their hospitals, without any thought about the welfare of the patients.

Government investigators found records showing that a homeless man was treated in an emergency room, then thrown out of the hospital because he was "filthy." He died on the hospital lawn.

Columbia/HCA executives were tried on charges of defrauding the government by systematically overstating the severity of illnesses they treated.

In the for-profit health care industry, business is business and profits have to come first or the business goes broke. For-profit HMOs were following the lead of hospitals and seeing themselves as businesses. Early on in the prepaid group practice-health maintenance organization movement the Group Health Association of America (GHAA) was formed to represent the groups then in existence, most of which were non-profit, like Kaiser Permanente and Health Insurance Plan of New York. Even Prudential was non-profit initially, but eventually it became for-profit, horrifying its many liberal-minded patrons. And Blue Cross, formed years before by hospitals to provide health insurance for Americans, began to split off for-profit subsidiaries. Eventually for-profits and not-for-profits diverged into two organizations.

GHAA was renamed American Association of Health Plans (AAHP) which initially was non-profit, but the realities of economics and politics forced AAHP to include commercial members and merge with the Health Insurance Association of America (HIAA) which was a cluster of for-profit insurance plans. But the constant movement of health insurance financing finally resulted in a newly named organization of for-profit and non-profit health plans called America's Health Insurance Plans (AHIP).

In 1999, after President Clinton asked that a prescription drug benefit be added to Medicare, the same big business-drug manufacturer coalition that destroyed catastrophic health insurance 12 years before swung into action. Their super expensive advertising campaign featured Flo, the senior citizen, reciting the same complaints that Harry and Louise had delivered for the commercial health insurance companies in 1993-94.

The plan was the same: fool people into thinking the big bad government is going to tarnish their lives and urge them to contact their Congressmen.

The lesson was: make money or else. The fateful development of managed care as a for-profit business was as natural as the stock market pages. As HMOs initially showed some promise as brakes on health care costs, the government—both Congressional and Executive branches—saw a great promise to save money for already rocketing costs of Medicare and Medicaid: encourage managed care insurers to lure beneficiaries and urge the beneficiaries to join for better savings and better service.

Immediately, as the Department of HHS and its Health Care Financing Administration developed plans to move beneficiaries of Medicare into managed care, managed care investors and administrators sought to keep costs down to make plans profitable and inviting for members.

But HMOs and hospitals are dealing with human lives and when costs get too big ambitious managers must think about the unthinkable—lower quality. The government has to pay no matter what. Doctors see this as their own judgments are questioned and patients see it through the diminished care they receive.

Some state health officials have reported rapidly growing numbers of formal complaints from both patients and doctors against health insurers.

"HMOs are targeting the doctors," a young emergency physician in Miami, Fla., omplained. "I can't give the tests I want in order to treat patients as I learned. All the HMOs care about is the cost."

In 1999, the Henry J. Kaiser Family Foundation, a study group founded with the fortunes of Kaiser Permanente but basically unbiased, reported that surveys showed almost nine out of ten doctors said their patients had experienced health plan denials of coverage for health services over the previous two years.

Eventually, being businesses, HMOs began making cutbacks. In the Washington, DC area in October of 1998, the Washington Post reported that "tens of thousands of patients…mostly senior citizens, must scramble to replace their health benefits over the next three months amid an exodus of managed care companies from Medicare."

This was particularly devastating to the idea of managed care as the open market competition solution since it was happening under the eyes of the entire federal government: Congress, HHS, the Defense Department and the Federal Employees Health Benefits Program (FEHB).

The HMOs were giving up because, they cried like a Greek chorus, the government wasn't paying them enough. The very principle of commercial managed care as the ideal free market business answer to government health insurance was collapsing.

"Consumers have sacrificed choice and now incur greatly increased bureaucratic impediments, but they have gained a system that is more accountable and provides incentives for integrated care," Arnold Epstein said in closing a Harvard School of Public Health report on managed care. “It should give them better care overall,” he concludes. “Maybe it will, maybe.”

Bill Bradley's Long Shot Misses

When former Sen. Bill Bradley (D-NJ) announced in 1997 that he was going to run for president of the United States, the press went wild. Here was the sort of story that sells newspapers and magazines: A Hall of Fame professional basketball star, high school and college basketball star and scholar, a Rhodes Scholar like Bill Clinton, a two-term U.S. Senator who had served with distinction on the coveted Senate Finance Committee and husband of a German-born intellectual who had survived a threatening bout with breast cancer.

Beginning with a colorful cover story in the nationally circulated Parade magazine, a seemingly endless stream of positive stories rolled out. The Washington Post ran a series of richly detailed stories about Bill Bradley the boy, the scholar, the athlete and the man. (Other candidates got this treatment later but Bradley was the first and clearly the most fun.) The Chicago Tribune ran a commentary by David Warsh of the Boston Globe headlined "Bradley could be a slam dunk as a candidate for the presidency." The story added, "Gore is almost certainly unelectable. His partnership with Clinton saddles him with too much baggage."

Even the Wall Street Journal's political triggerman Al Hunt wrote a favorable piece. Bill Bradley was the kind of guy everyone wanted—attractive, capable, not a hint of scandal around him. It was a long time before anyone could come up with any sort of negative story.

When they did it involved not a scandal but the "revelation" that he had a history of rapid heartbeats, not exactly crippling. Immediately, as is the case in our wired society, polls showed that Bradley was widely admired and ahead of his potential rival for the Democratic nomination, Vice President Al Gore. Then when Bradley said he was going to make health care one of his leading issues the political establishment took note. Both Gore and leading Republican candidate George W. Bush all of a sudden began talking about health care policy, which had been on the back shelf.

Although he had grabbed hold of an attractive issue, Bradley unfortunately began to illustrate his lack of skill as a political strategist and shot himself in the foot.

Many of the people he had conferred with on health policy advised against formulating a specific plan that could be riddled by enemy fire as the Clinton plan was. Bradley was having none of that. He announced to the world early on that he would present a plan that would be "raw meat." He meant to excite the electorate by detailing exactly how he would achieve what health policy philosophers had been calling the impossible task.

Former Congressional Budget Office director Robert Reischauer said that when Bradley called him for advice he recommended against a detailed plan. Reischauer said he asked, "Why do you need it?" and the candidate answered, "The press."

The candidate was making the worst mistake a politician can make. He was making his own press policy without expert advice, an interesting maneuver since as a Senator and member of the Finance Committee his press relations were notoriously uncooperative.

The fact that health care caught on early as a political issue was interpreted by experts as saying that a new administration could do what the Clintons failed to do: capitalize on what appeared to be an electoral mandate and make national health care happen.

Bradley did take one lesson from the Clinton mistake by avoiding anything like the often derided Hillary Clinton/Magaziner committee of 500. Instead Bradley carefully recruited a small but elite panel of top experts in health policy to help him assess the situation and formulate a pre-nomination proposal for a universal health care plan.

He assigned a former Senate aide, Margy Heldring, in whom he had great confidence, to organize the health plan. A psychologist, she interviewed experts and put together a plan that would insure that "no American has to worry about being one serious illness or injury away from financial ruin." The plan would have guaranteed health care for children then moved on to adults and senior citizens, who would have been granted drug coverage in addition to Medicare.

In order to move the poor from the Medicaid plan that many in the low income ranks feel is socially demeaning, Bradley suggested that they be covered by a voucher plan similar to the Federal Employees Health Benefits program. In describing this idea, Bradley noted that Medicaid eventually would be replaced, something, actually, that the Clinton-Gore plan would also have done.

But when the Bradley proposal was aired, his opponents, like the Vice President, immediately looked for something to criticize. A front-row Gore backer—a White House health adviser—seized on the idea of replacing Medicaid and began calling lobbyists and reporters to tell them Bradley was scrapping Medicaid, which the poor sick needed so desperately. Gore seized the fallacious criticism as a weapon to wound Bradley in their next television debate.

When Bradley was not able to counter the debating point, Gore continued to wield it. The telling venom of Gore's attack and Bradley's lack of debating skills to counter it fed the press with headline worthy stories, and Bradley's downward slide in the polls began.

Eventually, although he had vowed to fight hard for a health care plan and the nomination, he chose to give up and drop out. It was a sad end to a candidacy that had begun so well. Bradley had the lessons of history from the Clinton fiasco before him, but he didn't use them. He quit with a sizeable number of Democratic convention delegates he had won in the primaries, even though he had less than a working majority.

The lesson remained for ambitious candidates: health care is a major issue of interest to every American in one way or another. Bradley saw the appeal of health care as a campaign policy and determined early on to do something about it. But the negative forces that had prevented anything from happening earlier were there waiting for the next act and had already begun to make themselves evident. The commercial health insurance industry, for instance, already had begun to make new Harry and Louise commercials for radio and television.

Veteran observers concluded that the famous (or infamous) couple and their litany of complaints would be a permanent fixture in American politics.

Kennedy-Nixon

After passage of health insurance programs for the elderly and the poor, it was only a matter of time before public groups, organized labor and liberals in particular, were galvanized by the apparent need for health insurance for all. The first organized public move was made by one of the nation's outstanding healthcare advocates—Walter Reuther, head of the United Auto Workers Union. At the 1968 annual meeting of the American Public Health Association in Detroit, Reuther announced that he was setting up an organization to devise a plan and work for Congressional approval of it. He called the group the Committee of 100 for National Health Insurance. Original members of the 100 included philanthropist Mary Lasker who dynamically headed the national drive to expand the National Institutes of Health; heart surgeon Dr. Michael DeBakey, an ally of Mrs. Lasker; Whitney Young of the multi-racial Urban League, and others.

The CNHI, as it came to be known, set up a Washington office and national lobbying campaign. But first it needed a plan and a brain trust was set up to produce one. The authors included Dr. I.G. Falk, Yale University expert on government plans; Whitney Young; Vernon Jordan of the Urban League, and Bertrand Seidman, also of Urban.

The group came up with a plan called "Health Security." It would be financed by a trust fun with 40 percent coming from general tax revenues, 35 percent from a 1.8 percent employee tax on the first $15,000 of income. Providers would be paid according to prior budget estimates, and new group health plans would be developed.

A bill to put the plan into law was sponsored by Sen. Edward M. Kennedy (D-Mass) and Rep. Martha Griffiths (D-Mich). The proposal was met by vigorous opposition from the usual opponents of anything resembling a federal government plan. The AMA immediately called it socialized medicine and vowed opposition. Republicans in Congress were never enthusiastic and blocked committee action to the point where the bill never made it beyond meetings and speeches. Labor advocates in the meantime would have no part of compromising. In the words of an observer, organized labor demanded all or nothing at all, and nothing is what it got.

President Richard Nixon watched the Labor-Kennedy developments with great concern. Thinking of re-election prospects at the time, Nixon began work on a far-reaching NHI plan. In a November 1972 speech, he derided the Kennedy bill as meaning "government officials would have to approve hospital budgets and set fee schedules and take other steps that would eventually lead to the complete federal domination of American medicine."

Nixon, however, had made his own move by then. He sent Congress a Comprehensive Health Insurance Plan that would have required all employers to offer coverage to all full-time employees under age 65 through an insurance carrier that met basic standards set by the bill. A second part would have replaced most of Medicaid with an Assisted Health Insurance Plan.

The time was not right for Nixon or his plan, and it got nowhere. But, interestingly, in subsequent times it has not been unusual for experts to assess the plan as a good one that deserved consideration. The measure certainly had a powerful genesis. Authors of the bill were Nixon's chief health policy aides: James Cavanaugh, who would become a successful drug manufacturer executive and health industry consultant, as well as Paul O'Neill, Dick Cheney and Donald Rumsfeld who became, respectfully, George W. Bush's Treasury Secretary, Vice President and Defense Secretary.

President Jimmy Carter led his planners to another proposed national plan that sparked considerable debate before it, too, ran afoul of the standing army of negative forces.

Now What?

As the national health care issue entered the 21st century an increasingly bitter political debate continued over what to do about the uninsured—the unemployed young, the under-insured elderly who cannot afford the often great expenses that accompany aging, even with Medicare, and the poor in general.

Proposals abound, but any hope for a final solution, as it were, continues to be centered on the political and professional self-interests that have heretofore prevented any useful or promising proposals from maturing into law. Popular proposals range from Medicare for all to federal subsidies for private, for-profit health insurance. Where the ideas come from is very clear. More or less liberal Democrats of the school that produced Social Security and Medicare hold that Medicare works for the elderly and would be equally as useful for the younger with a federal financing system.

The answer lies between these people and conservatives who want for-profit entrepreneurs to handle the whole thing with funds moving from taxpayer-consumers through the federal government to the commercial interests. AMA, the commercial insurance business and conservatives who think Adam Smith had the answer have supported tax credit schemes as a device to avoid hated earmarked taxes and to encourage consumers to, in effect, pay their own bills without government interference or control.

Advocates of for-profit plans point out that even non-profit hospitals, for instance, are always concerned about profits from their operations. But what these critics don't say is that the non-profits want profits to improve their systems or to deliver charity care, particularly through emergency rooms where a lot of unpriced care takes place.

A favorite conservative plan is Medical Savings Accounts. This plan, sold for a time by the Golden Rule Insurance Co. Would set up a system where individuals regularly invest money in a putative savings account which would theoretically be left alone until there are medical bills to pay. The practicality of this idea reminds me of the time I started an auto savings plan to pay for my next car before I bought it. That lasted until I needed a new roof on my house.

MBAs were authorized in the 2003 legislation that established a controversial Medicare drug plan. In backing and making the law, conservatives said they were trying to improve Medicare and cut its costs. But it became clear that in advocating the Medicare "advancements" and, for that matter, demanding that Social Security be privatized, President George W. Bush was pandering to conservatives who want nothing more than to kill these New Deal and Fair Deal programs which a typical speaker from the Cato Institute or the Heritage Foundation will characterize as "a slippery slope" toward Socialism.

Also, the idea of Medicare for all is occasionally embellished by what some think should be the next chapter of Medicare—long term care (LTC). Long term care insurance is advised emphatically by financial and medical planners to prepare for what can be the disastrous expenses of nursing home or similar care for the elderly infirm. Some think it would be workable to add LTC premiums of a sort to Medicare taxes. At least all sides face the reality—that long term care is a problem that just about everyone has to face.

In the opinion of the author, any national health plan must be federally based. Introduction of private enterprise plans only opens the door to excesses like those that have plagued HMOs since they began moving toward the for-profit mode. Federal-State solutions are sometimes popular. Many conservative politicians would like to see the entire question handed to the states to handle with limited federal support. (This writer who covered civil rights in the South during critical years is aware of how the states individually handle matters.) The scourge of inflationary medical malpractice lawsuits and resultant high insurance prices is a matter which states, with the exception of California, have left largely untouched.

Probably the most important element that NHI requires, in addition to financing and universality, is equality. The efforts of insurers to keep costs of medical care down have contributed to a near national epidemic of medical errors. Certainly there is a terrible spate of medical malpractice today, as defined by the National Academy of Sciences' Institute of Medicine. But even those practitioners who are exceedingly careful find themselves constantly threatened by legal tricksters looking for patients they can persuade to seek profits when all they have suffered is bad luck.

In fact, one facet of medical cost inflation is the use of frequent expensive tests by doctors practicing defensive medicine to avoid being targeted by trial attorneys.

A federal plan with strong provisions of peer oversight by professional panels that would pass on the merits of litigation may be the answer.

The answer to the problem of the millions of uninsured could be a federal program modeled after Medicare or, perhaps, the highly regarded health plan lawmakers and government bureaucrats have fashioned for themselves. A plan like Medicare could cover basic costs of medical care while employers or individuals could purchase supplemental plans that many Medicare enrollees have. Or such "catastrophic" coverage could be made available reasonably by non-profit plans like Kaiser Permanente and the Blues used to be. Individuals could be helped in paying for the plans with the tax credits that Republicans long have supported. How terribly ironic it is that this country once had a catastrophic plan that would have taken care of drug costs for the elderly and which could have paved the road toward a similar plan for all as a supplement to a national plan for everyone.

It is necessary and possible. Wouldn't it be wonderful if an administration found the nation's health as vital as war on conceived sources of terrorism? What this country needs is another FDR or LBJ to take the lead in the public interest.